The interior of a late Victorian chemist's shop. This was Mr Castelow's shop in Woodhouse Lane, Leeds, and has been reconstructed at the Wilberforce House museum in Hull.

THE VICTORIAN CHEMIST AND DRUGGIST

W. A. Jackson

Shire Publications Ltd

CONTENTS

Set in 10 on 9 point Times roman and printed in Great Britain by C. I. Thomas & Sons (Haverfordwest) Ltd, Press Buildings, Merlins Bridge, Haverfordwest.

COVER: *Specie jar, cobalt blue syrup bottle with recessed glass label, wooden powder folder, pale blue glass eyebath.*

ACKNOWLEDGEMENTS

The author offers his thanks and gratitude to: his wife, Audrey, for her unfailing help and encouragement; Doctor John F. Wilkinson for his assistance and interest over many years, and for permission to photograph the leech jars, bench balance and blue and white infant feeding bottles from his collection; Manchester Public Libraries for permission to reproduce the illustration of Jewsbury and Brown's shop (page 3); City of Kingston upon Hull Museums and Art Galleries for permission to reproduce the photograph of the chemist's shop at Wilberforce House (page 1); the Société Jersiaise for permission to reproduce the photograph of the pharmacy display at the Jersey Museum (page 5). Other photographs are by Michael Bass of Lime Tree Studio, Tring.

Price and Company's shop (c 1810). Many large chemist and druggist's shops would have looked like this at the start of Victoria's reign. Note the small panes of glass and the storage vessels on display.

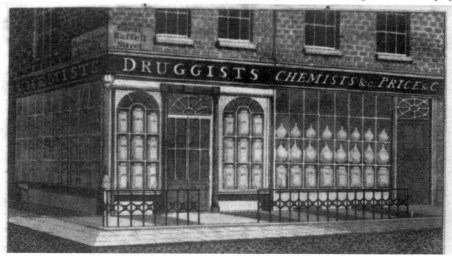

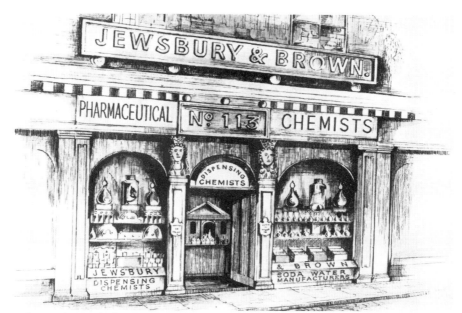

Jewsbury and Brown's shop (late nineteenth century). Each window is a single large sheet of glass and contains goods for sale with the specie jars and display carboys above.

INTRODUCTION

In 1617 the apothecaries, who were a well defined group of the Grocers' Company, separated from them to form the Society of Apothecaries, a Livery Company of the City of London which is still in existence. They kept open shop, giving advice and supplying medicines to patients who could not afford to consult a physician. In the eighteenth century there was a tendency for them to split into two groups, those who were to become general practitioners and those who dispensed medicines, and by 1775 'trading' apothecaries could no longer become liverymen of the Society.

The merging of the chemists (dealers in chemicals) and the druggists (who dealt in drugs of animal and vegetable origin) to become chemists and druggists was a gradual process which was well established by the end of the eighteenth century, and in 1815 their right to buy, compound, dispense and sell drugs and medicines by wholesale or retail was established by Act of Parliament. During the nineteenth century they were joined by the 'trading' apothecaries, giving rise to the Victorian chemist and druggist.

In 1841 the Pharmaceutical Society of Great Britain was formed, and in 1852 a register of chemists and druggists, associates and students was set up, and the Society given power to examine persons for registration. The Pharmacy Act of 1868 introduced Schedules of Poisons and a higher qualification, the pharmaceutical chemist. Only pharmaceutical chemists and chemists and druggists (registration of both being dependent on examination) were allowed to supply poisons from the First Schedule to the public. The number of pharmaceutical chemists was small compared with the chemists and druggists, and the latter remained the main supplier of medicines and associated articles to the nation.

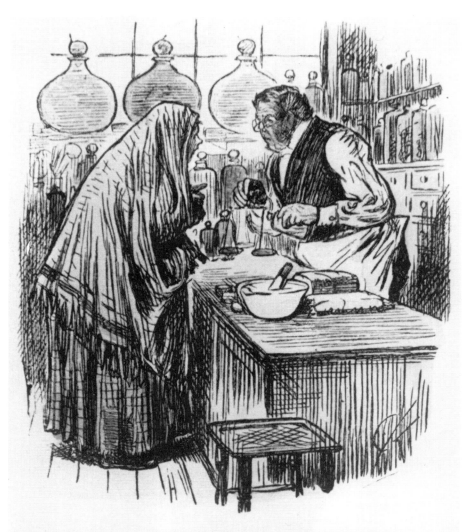

"AGAINST THE GRAIN"

Widow Woman (to Chemist, who was weighing a grain of calomel in dispensing a prescription for her sick child). " Man, ye needna' be sae scrimpy wi't—'tis for a puir fatherless bairn ! "

The interior of a small shop. The proprietor is using a handscale. The drug run can be seen behind the counter.

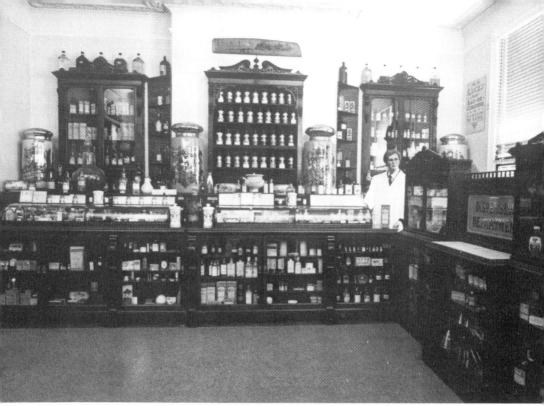

The interior of a St Helier pharmacy (late nineteenth century), reconstructed in the Jersey Museum. Medicines, perfumery and sundries are displayed in glass-fronted cases and on top of the counter, but the shelves are still occupied by shop rounds.

THE SHOP

At the start of Victoria's reign the majority of shops had windows which were made up of panes of glass 12 by 16 inches (305 by 406 mm) in size. They were normally used as extensions of storage shelving and held containers of the drugs which were sold or used in dispensing. Although these containers were often of poor quality, the labelling made many of them quite decorative, and the overall effect must have been attractive. They must also have been useful in identifying the type of shop to a population that was largely illiterate. It is

thought that shortly before this time jars of water-white glass holding coloured liquids began to be displayed for this purpose. As time went on, large show carboys and elaborately decorated specie jars replaced the earlier crude glass containers.

In the 1830s plate glass was introduced, and there was a gradual change from the old type of window to one composed of (usually) three large panes. This type of window lent itself to the display of products such as patent medicines and began to be used in this way to promote impulse buying. By 1900 larger sheets of plate glass were available, and many shop windows consisted of a single sheet, behind which were displayed the chemist's own remedies, patent medicines, toiletries and articles used in the sickroom. Surmounting this display were the carboys or specie jars which were now the acknowledged sign of the chemist and druggist.

Inside, the focal point of the shop was the counter. This usually held a brass beamscale on which drugs were weighed for sale. In many small shops it also served as the dispensing bench, although this became less common as time went on. Usually a screen was erected along part of the counter, and dispensing operations were carried out behind this, but in larger shops a separate room in the rear of the premises was converted for this purpose.

Another important feature was the drug run. This was a set of drawers with wooden knobs and painted labels (later ones often had glass knobs and painted and gilded glass labels). The drawers held herbs, roots, powdered chemicals and so on. Above this were shelves of bottles or earthenware jars. As sales of articles other than medicines became a significant part of the business, glass showcases in which they could be displayed became increasingly important. The fittings were usually of solid mahogany, which was kept well polished. Labour was cheap and working hours were long, many shops remaining open until 10 or 11 pm. The chemist presided over the counter, the cleaning, routine jobs and much of the dispensing being done by apprentices or assistants, who normally wore long aprons.

Large storage vessels. (Left to right) Two early bottles, the one for rose water relabelled in the second half of the century; large unlabelled bottle 21½ inches (580 mm) high; small specie jar; pear-shaped storage carboy (c 1850); round storage carboy (late eighteenth or early nineteenth century).

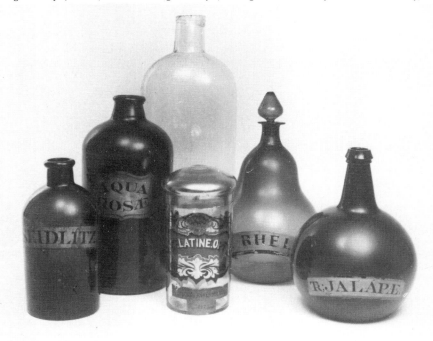

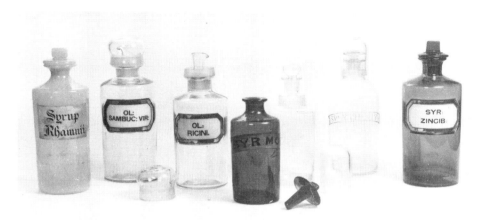

Shop rounds. (Left to right) Rare pale blue opaque syrup bottle with paper label; two oil bottles with recessed glass labels; early cobalt blue syrup bottle painted label; two aether rounds (one with engraved label); cobalt blue syrup bottle with recessed glass label.

STORAGE CONTAINERS

As we have seen, many dry drugs were kept in drawers, but with frequently used items this was only a working stock, the drawers being refilled from bulk which was stored in barrels or sacks. Another type of container was the glass *specie jar*. These were painted and gilded on the inside with elaborate scrollwork or a coat of arms as well as the name of the contents. They varied in height from about $10\frac{1}{2}$ inches (280 mm) to 31 inches (770 mm) and they were frequently displayed in the shop window. Smaller quantities of solids were kept in glass bottles known as *shop rounds* (so called because they were round in section) with wide necks.

Carboys and large glass bottles were the normal containers for liquids which were used in quantity. Smaller amounts were stored in shop rounds, which usually had ground glass stoppers, but there were some specialised types for different liquids. *Syrup bottles* were fitted with loose peg stoppers to avoid their being cemented in the neck of the bottle by crystallised sugar. Because they were loose, these stoppers usually had a wide flange to stop dust getting into the neck. *Oil bottles* had a special removable

lip for pouring and a reservoir round the neck of the bottle so that after use any drips would drain into this and then back into the bottle instead of running down the outside and on to the shelf. *Aether rounds* were used for volatile liquids. They had heavy glass domes over the stoppers so that if these were blown out in hot weather they merely hit the dome and dropped back into the neck of the bottle. During the course of Victoria's reign, as more and more drugs came into use, smaller quantities of each were kept, and the carboys and very large bottles were relegated to cellars or retained for decorative purposes only.

Most bottles were made of colourless glass, but cobalt blue was sometimes used, particularly for syrups, and actinic green glass was popular for poisons. With the advent of moulded bottles *poison rounds* were often made distinguishable to the touch, usually by being fluted vertically.

Bottles are not easily dated, as some glassworks continued to make them by hand long after others had changed to machine moulding. However, there are some guidelines. Early bottles usually have

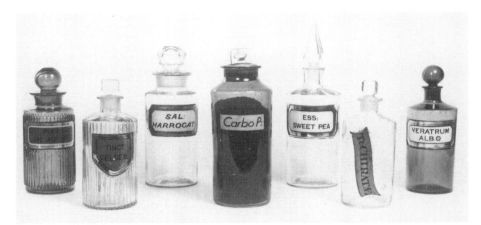

ABOVE: *Shop rounds. (Left to right) Fluted green poison with red recessed glass label; fluted white poison with red recessed shield label; round with faceted glass stopper; early round with rough pontil and hand-made stopper; perfume bottle with elegant stopper; round with painted ribbon label; green round with globe stopper.*

BELOW: *Storage jars. Four earthenware jars with paper, recessed glass and painted labels; moulded stoneware jar with japanned lid and painted label.*

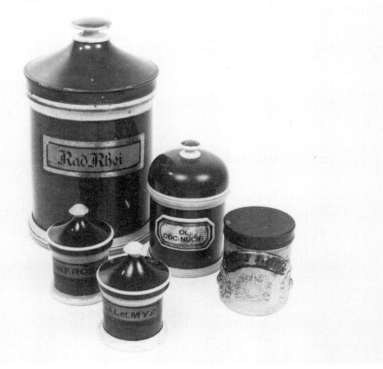

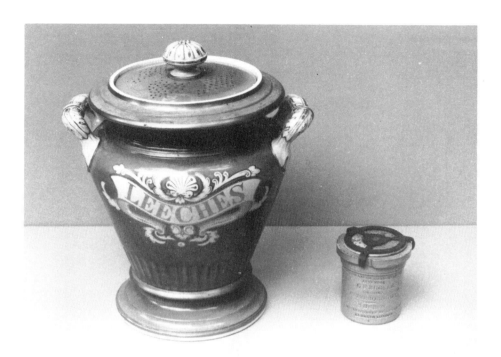

Leech jars. A large blue earthenware jar, and Buckle's 'leech conservatory' with a metal clip to hold the lid in place.

a rough pontil and a fairly high kick. In later hand-made specimens the pontil was often smoothed by grinding, and moulded bottles display marks where the separate pieces of the mould were joined. Most early labels were engraved or (more commonly) painted, but towards the end of the century bottles were moulded with recessed panels, and curved, rectangular glass labels with mitred corners were cemented into the recesses. Varnished handwritten paper labels were used throughout the whole period.

Creams and ointments were stored in earthenware or salt-glazed stoneware jars. The latter were often decorated with a design, such as the royal coat of arms,

moulded in relief. They were fitted with japanned tin covers, and, although these were sometimes used for the earthenware jars as well, the majority of the latter had matching earthenware lids which were either flat, domed or shaped like the top of a bell. This type of container was often used to hold dry drugs as well as ointments.

Live medicinal leeches, which were used to bleed people, were a normal item of stock, and specially made *leech jars* were available for them. These were usually of creamware or coloured earthenware, with flat or domed lids which were perforated to allow air to enter. Another type made in earthenware and stoneware had a lid which was held firmly in place by a metal clip.

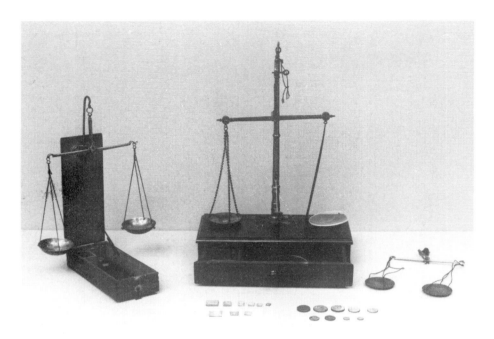

ABOVE: *Scales and weights. (Left to right) Portable boxed scale with swan-neck ends; bench balance with box ends; handscale with swan-neck ends. (Foreground) Rough square and well finished coin-shaped apothecary weights.*

BELOW: *Glass measures. Three conical measures graduated in fluid ounces and drachms, and a cylindrical measure graduated in drachms and minims.*

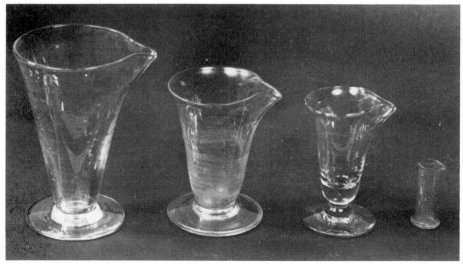

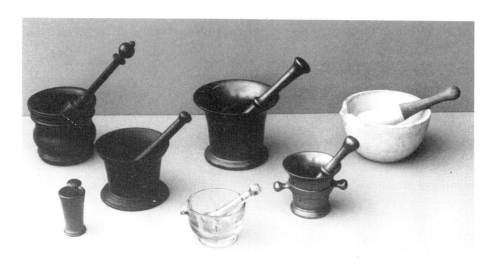

Mortars and pestles. (Left to right: back row) Lignum vitae, bell metal, composition; (centre) iron, brass; (front) boxwood, glass.

DISPENSING EQUIPMENT

Although the brass *beamscales* on the shop counter were used for fairly large quantities of powders, they were not sensitive enough for accurate measurement of the small amounts often required in dispensing. For this the commonest type used in the nineteenth century was the small, equal-arm *handscale* with swan-neck ends, but towards the end of the century they were gradually being replaced by *bench scales* with agate bearings, which were more accurate. Less commonly found are the portable bench scales which could be dismantled and stored in the boxes which supported them when in use. Apothecary, troy and avoirdupois *weights* were all in everyday use. Early examples are usually plain and roughly square in shape, but, from 1847 onwards, weights shaped like lozenges or coins were produced by W. and T. Avery and Rogers and Company. These were very successful despite the criticism that their embossed surface picked up and retained dirt.

Most of the *measures* used for liquids are conical, made from glass with engraved graduations, and may carry an etched verification stamp from which it is possible to date them. Translucent horn was another material used, but these are rather scarce. Copper and pewter measures were frequently used for larger quantities. Powders were often measured by volume instead of weight, and double cup measures of boxwood are quite common. Some of these were for specific purposes, such as the charges for Gazogene machines and the two powders used in Seidlitz powders.

Mortars and *pestles* were used for reducing lumpy or crystalline solids and dried herbs to a fine powder, as well as for bruising roots and rhizomes before extracting their active principles. They were made from many different materials such as bell metal, brass, iron, glass, ivory and hard woods such as lignum vitae or boxwood. One disadvantage of metal mortars was the danger of their reacting with the chemicals in them. This had led to Josiah Wedgwood investigating the possibility of using ceramic materials, and about 1780 he produced a substance which he called 'biscuit porcelain', which became widely used. Nowadays these are usually called *composition* mortars.

The simplest form of medicine dispensed

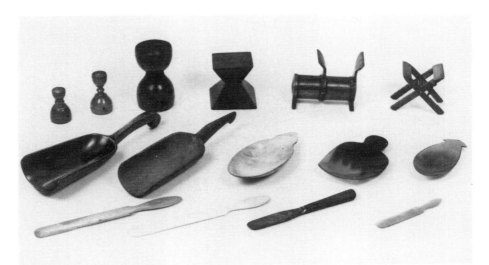

ABOVE: *Items used in making wrapped powders. (Left to right: back row) Three boxwood double powder measures; one wooden and two adjustable brass folders; (centre) two wooden and three horn scoops; (front) bone, metal and horn spatulae.*

BELOW: *Pillmaking equipment. Pill machine, graduated pill tile, double-ended mortar and pestle, boxwood silverer, porcelain pot for varnishing, boxwood rounder and pill spatula.*

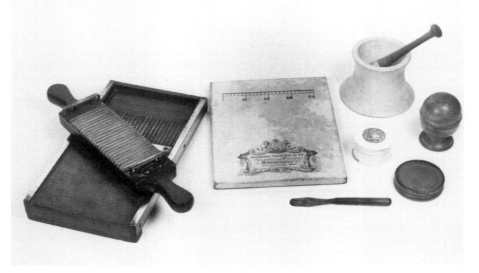

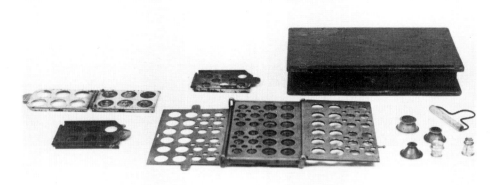

Cachet machines. Three primitive cachet machines (for different sizes of cachet), and a Morstadt cachet machine.

was the powder. All the ingredients were reduced to a fine powder by grinding in a mortar if necessary, the final mixing being done on a sheet of white paper with a spatula. The bulk powder was then divided into individual doses and wrapped by hand in sheets of pre-cut paper. The final folds were made on a *powder folder* (usually adjustable), so that when finished they were all of the correct length to fit snugly into the box in which the customer received them.

Powders had the disadvantage that many of them had an unpleasant taste. One way of overcoming this was to make them into pills. Usually, the active ingredients were mixed in a *pill mortar* with liquorice powder and just sufficient liquid glucose to form a firm but pliable mass. This was rolled into a *pipe* or cylinder of the required length, which could then be divided by means of a spatula on a graduated tile, the pills then being rounded between finger and thumb. Many dispensaries possessed *pill machines*. These were usually made of mahogany with brass runners and cutters. This was placed on a firm bench and the pipe rolled on the wooden baseboard. It was then placed on the lower brass grooves, the two-handled upper part of the cutter placed over it and pushed to and fro until the roughly spherical pills rolled into the open drawer at the back of the machine. In both cases the final shape was achieved by rolling the pills on a tile under

a boxwood or iron rounder. They were then allowed to harden, after which they were varnished. Finally, they were sometimes silvered or gilded by rotating them in a spherical boxwood container with silver or gold leaf and a little gum.

Another way of disguising the taste of powders was to place them between two pieces of rice paper. The edges were then moistened and would stick together. When placed on the tongue, the rice paper became soft and the entire 'wafer' could be swallowed. It was from these wafers that cachets were developed. In these, the rice paper was preformed into shapes similar to tiny soup plates. The powder was placed in one, the rim of another moistened and then pressed down on to the first one, forming the cachet, which was shaped rather like a flying saucer. In the latter part of the century *cachet machines* such as the Morstadt were developed, making filling and sealing much cleaner, easier and quicker.

Suppositories and *pessaries,* designed for insertion into the rectum and vagina respectively, contained medicaments in a base made from cocoa butter or glycerine and gelatine. The semi-molten mass was poured into moulds and allowed to cool and set. Suppositories were commonly conical with a rounded tip, and approximately 15 grains in weight, pessaries weighing 30 or 60 grains. Moulds for 120 grain pessaries are not uncommon, but these were usually for veterinary use. Nasal and

13

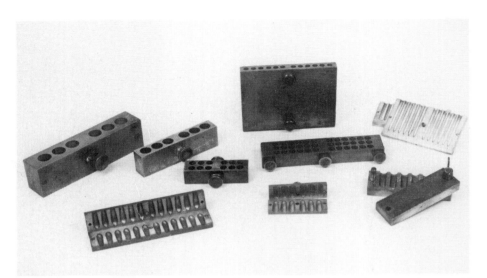

ABOVE: *Suppository, pessary and bougie moulds. One bougie mould and three suppository moulds are shown open.*

BELOW: *(Left to right) Cork press; set of brass cork borers; infusion pot; plaster iron and roll of lead plaster mass; cork press.*

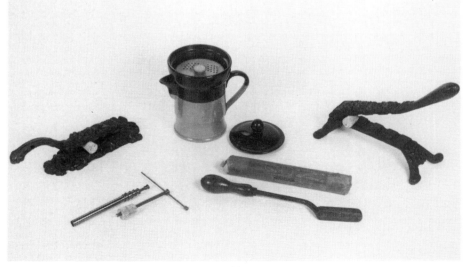

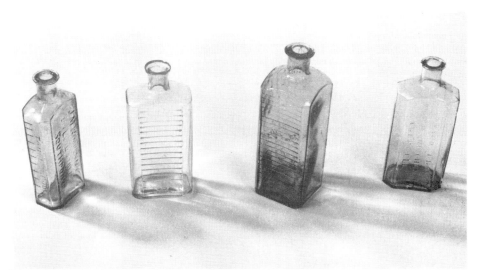

Dispensing bottles showing graduations or the name and address of the chemist. The left-hand bottle has both.

urethral *bougies* were medicated pencils prepared in the same way, but were thinner and longer, the commonest lengths being $2\frac{1}{2}$ inches (64 mm) and 4 inches (102 mm).

At the beginning of the nineteenth century, many liquid medicines for internal use were supplied in the form of a vial containing a single dose or draught. In Victoria's reign there was a rapid growth in the use of multi-dose bottles for medicines, and by the 1860s these accounted for much of the output of dispensed medicines. Many of these mixtures contained fresh infusions made from such things as dried bitter orange peel, cloves, gentian root, hops or senna. These were made by allowing the crude drugs to remain in contact with water (usually hot) for a definite period of time and then straining. It was found that if the drug was suspended near the surface of the liquid the active principles were extracted more efficiently, and this led to *infusion pots* being made with a removable perforated plate, on which the drug was placed, near the top of the vessel.

Plasters for external application were prepared extemporaneously. The in-gredients were mixed with a base of lead plaster (made from lead oxide, olive oil and water) or one made from a mixture of resin and soap. They were solid when cold but became flexible and adhesive at body temperature. They were spread by means of a hot *plaster iron* on pieces of sheepskin, chamois leather, calico, silk or swansdown (a thick cotton cloth with a soft nap on one side) which had previously been cut to the required size and shape.

Although most chemists and druggists bought bottles in a range of standard sizes, for which they had the correct corks, they also used bottles returned to them by customers, and these frequently had necks for which there were no suitable corks in stock. When this occurred, a cork which was slightly too large could be squeezed in a *cork press* until it was a good fit. A set of *cork borers* was usually kept to bore holes in corks to accommodate glass tubes of different diameters.

Medicine bottles were usually octagonal and might be graduated and have the name and address of the chemist moulded in the glass.

15

IF YOU COUGH

TAKE

GÉRAUDEL'S PASTILLES

(WHICH ACT BY INHALATION AND ABSORPTION DIRECTLY UPON THE RESPIRATORY ORGANS) FOR

**COUGHS,
COLDS,
INFLUENZA,
BRONCHITIS,
HOARSENESS,
CATARRH,
ASTHMA,
LARYNGITIS,
&c.**

*THEIR EFFECT IS
INSTANTANEOUS.*

Price per Case, 1/1½, with directions for use, of all Chemists, or will be sent post free on receipt of price from the WHOLESALE DEPOT FOR GREAT BRITAIN—

FASSETT & JOHNSON,
32, Snow Hill, London, E.C.

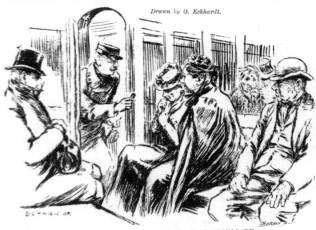

Drawn by O. Eckhardt.

THE UNDERGROUND RAILWAY—AS IT SHOULD BE.
GUARD (to choking and coughing female): "Here, take a Géraudel's Pastille and welcome! The company provides 'em. I've never been afraid of damp, fog, or cold since I carried a case of Géraudel's."

ABOVE: *Pictorial advertisement for Geraudel's cough pastilles.*

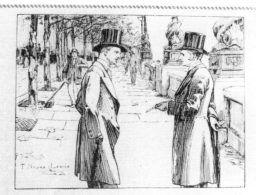

1st DOCTOR: "What time did that child die?"

2nd DOCTOR: "You will hardly believe it, but, thanks to 'Frame Food' Diet, it is still alive and thriving splendidly!"

The above refers to a baby suffering from Rickets, Inflammation of the Bowels, and Convulsions; no food stayed on its stomach, though several well-known foods were tried. The child's Doctor, and another called in to consult with him, pronounced the case hopeless. In despair the mother asked if nothing could be done to save the child's life; the Doctors said they feared not, but one Doctor suggested to try "Frame Food" Diet. This was done, and the child immediately improved, had no more Convulsions, and the sickness soon ceased.

LEFT: *Advertisement for patent food.*

16

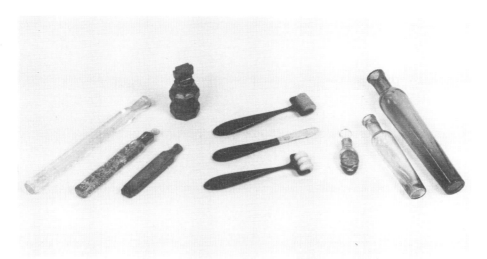

(Left to right) Three thick-walled perfume bottles; blue cut glass smelling salt bottle; two ivory and ebony massage roulettes and spatula; smelling salt bottle with original label; two late nineteenth-century perfume phials.

COUNTER LINES

Many chemists and druggists packed their own remedies and sold these together with nationally advertised patent medicines. Extravagant claims were made for many of the latter, and the introduction of pictorial advertising must have helped to increase their sales.

Similarly, they made their own perfumes in the dispensary (some such as 'Jockey Club' were made to standard formulae, while others were given local names such as 'Levenshulme Bouquet'), and these were sold as well as the products of firms like Yardley, Atkinson and Rimmel.

Toiletries included hair dressings and tonics (e.g. bears' grease and macassar oil), hair dyes and setting lotions, toilet powders, perfumed soaps, rouge, lip salves, cold cream and tooth powders and pastes. Again, many of these were made in the dispensary or bought in bulk and packed in containers bearing the name and address of the shop.

Infant and invalid foods were good sellers, and in addition to the things listed above most shops sold a great variety of household items one does not expect to find in the modern pharmacy. Sauces, pickles and spices, tea and cocoa, dyes, varnishes, ink, candles, lamp oil, wicks, matches, tobacco and aerated waters were all commonly stocked, and it was not unusual to find a section devoted to 'garden, flower and agricultural seeds'.

Until recently virtually all that remained to remind us of all this activity were some polychrome printed pot lids from jars that had originally contained bears' grease or toothpaste, a handful of ceramic advertising figures and the advertisements to be found in old magazines. Since 1970 however, the development of 'dump digging' as a hobby has produced a wealth of monochrome printed jars and pot lids (many of them very local in distribution) and old medicine bottles from the Victorian rubbish dumps in which they had lain undisturbed since their original owners threw them away. Most of the bottles originally had paper labels, and it is no longer possible to identify their erstwhile contents, but the jars and pot lids reveal the great variety of both local and national products which had been packed in this way. Although not as attractive in appearance as the polychrome lids, these are often of greater importance to those interested in local history.

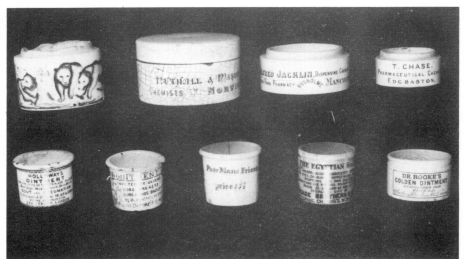

ABOVE: *Ointment pots. (Top row) Bears' grease; pots used for packing chemist's own products. (Bottom) Proprietary ointments.*
BELOW: *Pot lids for bears' grease, cold creams and toothpastes.*

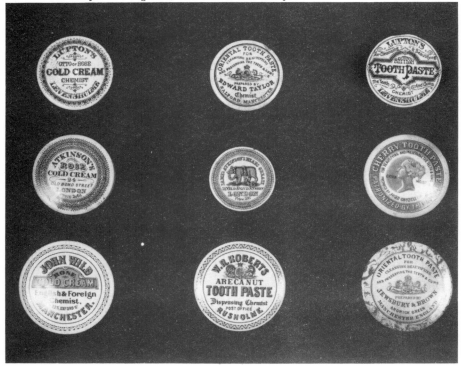

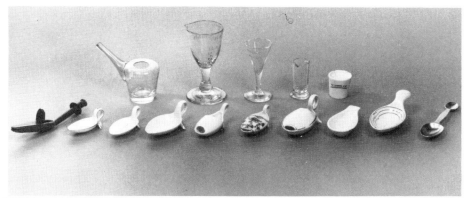

Medicine measures and spoons. (Left to right: back row) Unusual spouted glass measure; two 'wineglass' measures and one cylindrical glass measure; earthenware measure; (front) pewter Gibson spoon; three open medicine spoons; three with half-covers; two with graduations for tea, dessert and table spoons; silver double-ended salt and tea spoon (1888).

CHEMISTS' SUNDRIES

Another important part of the stock was known collectively as chemists' sundries, consisting mainly of articles used in the sickroom or nursery.

With an increasing number of medicines being supplied in multi-dose bottles, the use of *medicine spoons* was already well established by 1837. Probably the commonest type was of earthenware or porcelain, with a looped rear handle and two small leaf-like feet. Sometimes the bottom of the bowl was flattened to ensure greater stability and some had half-covers. One disadvantage was the variation in the size of their bowls, and by the middle of the 1870s spoons were available which were graduated for tea, dessert and table spoons. Another spoon, designed for the administration of unpleasant medicine to 'fractious children or to insane persons', was first publicly demonstrated by its inventor, Charles Gibson, in 1828, and soon achieved widespread popularity. These were commonly made of pewter but are also known in silver, Britannia metal and porcelain. Other spoons, often double-ended, were made of silver or plated metal. *Measures* were normally made of earthenware or glass. Some were for a single dose, but others were graduated.

There are some attractive glass measures shaped like lipped wine glasses with engraved graduations, those of earthenware usually being conical or bucket-shaped with internal markings. An unusual type of hand-made glass measure had a spout and was particularly useful for administering medicine to patients who were unable to sit up.

The Victorians were great travellers, and the more affluent often carried their own *medicine cabinets*, particularly when going abroad. These were supplied by many of the larger chemists and druggists and usually contained bottles of medicaments, a hand balance, weights, measure, mortar and pestle, and a booklet of formulae for medicines to treat common complaints. Most of those to be found nowadays are incomplete, and it is rare indeed to find one with its original booklet. They are usually known as *apothecaries' cabinets* in the antique trade.

For those who regularly took one particular medicine, *cased bottles* were available. These were made from the 1840s onwards, the bottle being protected from the rigours of travel by a wooden case. Most of these were made of boxwood, but rosewood and ebony were also used.

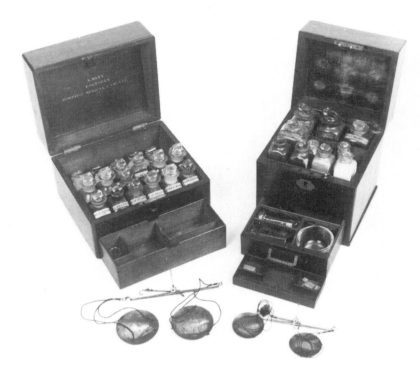

Domestic medicine cabinets. (Left) A removable tray holds scales and a minim measure, and there is a glass slab for mixing ointments behind a flap in the lid. (Right) The scales and weights are in a tray in the drawer, which also holds a measure and small glass mortar and pestle.

Although nearly all were designed for liquid medicines, it is possible to find wide-mouthed bottles for carrying powders. Boxes were also made to hold toilet powders, and one can still find them with their original swansdown puffs. Farr's Patent Ampulla was a boxwood container for tooth powder which was patented in 1865. It was designed to keep the powder dry and was claimed to be economical because one could sprinkle the powder on to the brush instead of dipping wet bristles into it.

Chest complaints were then, as now, very common and most shops would have in stock such things as *bronchitis kettles,* inhalers and sputum mugs. The kettles were used as a source of steam to ease lung congestion. The patient sat in a tent made of bedsheets, and the spout of the kettle was introduced into this. The purpose of the long neck was to keep the source of heat well away from the sheets to obviate the risk of fire. The Nelson *inhaler,* which is still in use today, was introduced in the nineteenth century but differed from modern specimens in having a blue marbled body and a mouthpiece made of thick glass, which was held firmly in the neck of the inhaler by a cork shim and contained a small piece of natural sponge. Nowadays, this has been replaced by a flat cork through which a bent glass tube passes. Aromatics, such as friars' balsam, were mixed with hot water in the bulbous body, and the resulting vapour was inhaled through the mouthpiece. *Sputum mugs* contained water into which the patient could spit to get rid of phlegm. The contents were concealed from view by a funnel

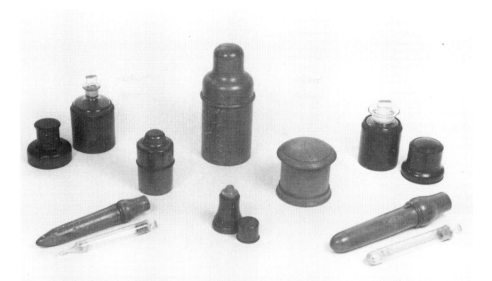

ABOVE: *Three bottles for liquids in boxwood cases; one for powder in an ebony case; a box for toilet powder; two syringes in boxwood cases; and a boxwood container for tooth powder (Farr's Patent Ampulla).*
BELOW: *A copper bronchitis kettle and three Nelson inhalers with thick glass mouthpieces.*

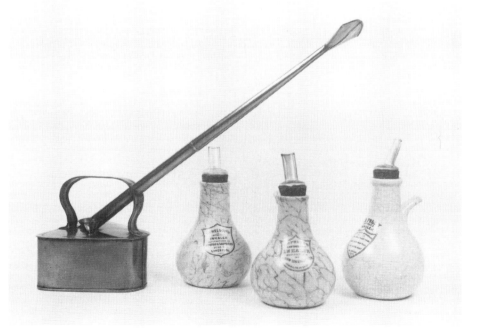

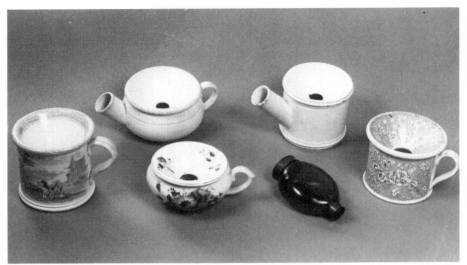

Sputum mugs and bottle. (Back row) Two white earthenware mugs with integral funnels and hollow handles for emptying. (Front) Mugs with removable funnels, two with blue transfer and one with polychrome decoration; a blue glass sputum bottle with pewter caps at top and bottom.

in the top of the mug. In many early specimens this was an integral part of the mug, the contents being emptied through a hollow side handle. Later on, removable funnels were introduced to facilitate their emptying and cleaning. Many were decorated with blue transfer prints or a floral pattern. *Sputum bottles,* usually of blue glass with pewter caps, were designed to be carried in the pocket or reticule.

Many Victorians were greatly concerned with the regular evacuation of their bowels. By the 1830s the large pewter *enema syringe* or *clyster,* which had been much favoured by physicians in the eighteenth century, had to a great extent been replaced by a simple rubber bulb which was attached to a bone nozzle. An important development in the history of the enema was the invention of a two-way syringe with ball valves by John Read. This proved to be very popular and was widely copied by other makers, remaining in use for many years. Later in the century, syringes with sheet metal reservoirs which could be used without the assistance of a second person were produced. The patient sat down on the upright nozzle and depressed the piston which went down into the reservoir. These were dangerous machines, and

the hard nozzles must have been responsible for many injuries, while the jet produced was sufficiently strong to strip the rectal mucosa.

Bedpans of circular shape with a hollow side handle are known to have been in use from the sixteenth century and remained popular throughout Victoria's reign. Both the pewter and the brown glazed earthenware specimens illustrated tended to be superseded by bedpans of similar shape, but made from white glazed earthenware, as the century progressed. The 1830s saw the introduction of the 'Slipper' bedpan. This revolutionary design was a great advance, being much easier to use when the patient was unable to sit upright in bed. The 'Shovel,' which was in use by the 1860s, proved to be a poor competitor, possibly because, despite the hollow handle, it was more difficult to empty and clean.

Urinals are found in a number of different shapes, but the commonest one is oval with a flattened base and extended neck. Those intended for male use have a circular opening, whereas those with a flared or oval mouth are for females. They were commonly made from white glazed earthenware, but examples in glass (rarely

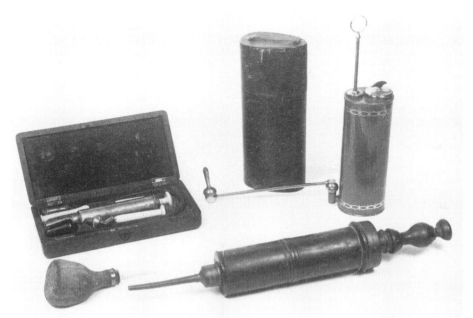

ABOVE: *Enema syringes. A cased pewter and bone syringe of the type designed by John Read; a rubber bulb with bone nozzle; a syringe with sheet metal reservoir; a pewter clyster with wooden piston — length 18 inches (450 mm).*
BELOW: *Bedpans. 'Slipper' bedpan; round brown glazed earthenware with hollow handle; pewter with handle which unscrews; 'Shovel' with curved hollow handle.*

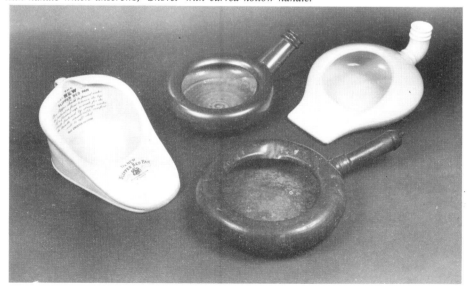

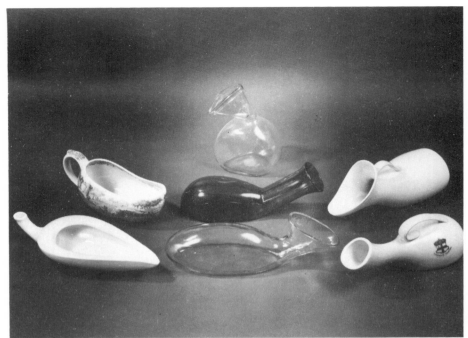

ABOVE: *Urinals. (Left to right: back) Glass upright female; (middle) bourdalou; blue glass male; earthenware female with flattened end so that it can be stood upright after use; (bottom) spoonbill; glass female; earthenware male.*

BELOW: *Hand-made glass eyebaths. Note the bath with a reservoir (fourth from left).*

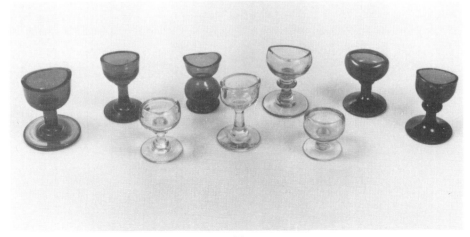

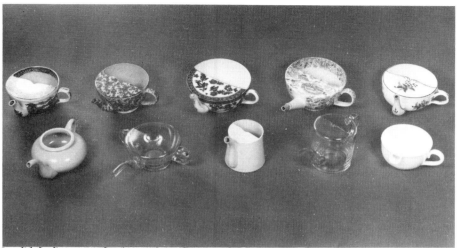

Invalid feeding cups showing various shapes and types of decoration.

cobalt blue) are to be found. Upright urinals with a flask-shaped or roughly triangular body were also made in glass or earthenware. Another type of female urinal was the open boat-shape, which was sometimes narrower in the middle, giving it a slight figure of eight outline. These were known as bourdalous, another English name for them being coach pots (from their being carried in stage coaches for the relief of passengers during long journeys). They were often decorated with blue transfer prints and are eagerly sought by collectors. The spoonbill was yet another type of urinal intended for female use. It was flat and roughly triangular in shape, having a pipe-like opening at the broad end through which it could be emptied.

The majority of Victorian *eyebaths* which one finds nowadays are made from glass, usually colourless or in varying shades of blue or green, although other colours are to be seen occasionally. Typically, they consist of a foot, a stem (which may be knopped) and a bowl. The rim of the bowl was usually flamed after cutting to smooth the sharp edges and was sometimes turned inwards while the glass was still soft. One sometimes finds examples in which the rim was smoothed by grinding instead of flaming. Eyebaths were

also made from silver, base alloys and ceramic materials; but interesting specimens are usually very expensive. Baths in which the stem is replaced by a more or less spherical reservoir may be found, although relatively few of them seem to have survived.

Anyone who has tried to drink from an ordinary cup while lying flat on his back will appreciate the advantage of a *feeding cup* in the sickroom. These were available in a variety of shapes, but those with a hemispherical bowl with a flat half-cover and a handle to the right of a straight or curved spout enjoyed the greatest popularity. This shape is also found with a rear handle, one at each side of the spout, three handles, or (rarely) one to the left of the spout. They were frequently decorated, usually with blue transfer prints of landscapes or flowers. In one type the spout is replaced by a lip; another is shaped like a small teapot, and a third (without a handle) is reminiscent of shapes which were more popular in the eighteenth century. Feeding cups made of glass are more fragile than ceramic ones and fewer have survived, while examples in silver or pewter are scarce.

Food warmers or *veilleuses* were in common use throughout the nineteenth century.

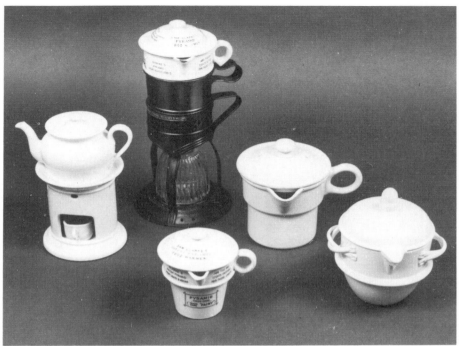

Tea warmer, food warmer and pannikins. The pannikins originally had metal stands, but earlier ones had ceramic stands similar to that of the tea warmer.

They usually consisted of a hollow pedestal which held a godet or lamp (originally an earthenware vessel containing oil and a wick, later replaced by a night light), and a lidded pannikin for the food. Towards the end of the century, the ceramic pedestals were replaced by ones made from metal, and the pannikin rested on a container of hot water known as a liner. They were often used to prepare a mixture of flour or bread with diluted milk which was called pap and used for feeding infants — hence the alternative name of *pap warmer*. Some were intended for preparing herbal teas, and in these the pannikin was replaced by a teapot, the apparatus then being known as a *tea warmer* or *veilleuse tisanniere*.

Pap was used extensively for feeding infants and was usually given by means of a

pap boat. These were small boat-shaped vessels, the earlier examples being open with one end drawn into a lip. Later, a half-cover was added, the lip becoming a spout. This type usually had a small fan-shaped handle at the back, which became a loop in those made towards the end of the century. With the decline in the use of pap as a baby food, many wholesalers began to list their pap boats as invalid feeders, and large numbers of long-spouted cups with looped rear handles were made which were too large to be intended for use as pap boats. Open boats were often decorated with blue transfer designs, while those with half-covers usually had multicoloured flowers, often hand-painted. Also known, but less easily found, are pap boats made from silver, pewter, glass and wood.

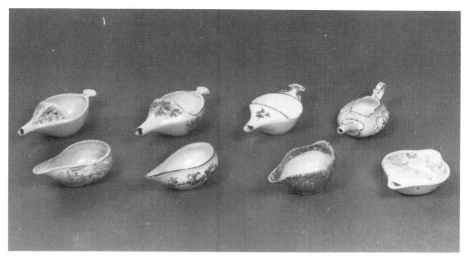

ABOVE: *Pap boats used for feeding infants, showing different shapes and types of decoration.*

BELOW: *Pewter and earthenware infant feeding bottles.*

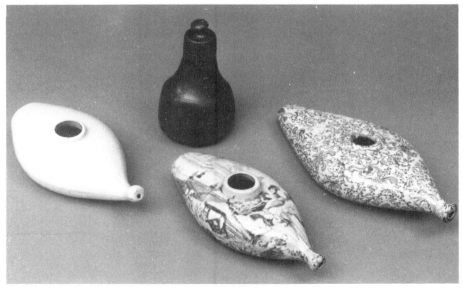

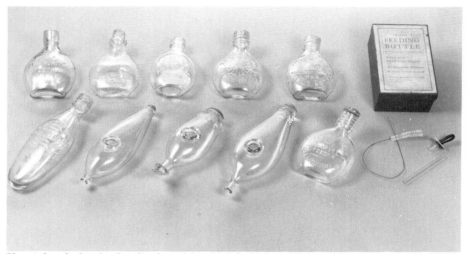

Glass infant feeding bottles. (Back row) Moulded flask-shaped bottles. (Front) Long moulded bottle; three hand-made bottles; moulded bottle with its original box, brush, glass tube, shield and teat (rubber tubing missing).

Although their heyday was over, pear-shaped pewter *feeding bottles* were still used throughout the reign of Victoria. Earthenware bottles with a hole in the upper side, through which they were filled, were a fairly recent innovation. Most were made in Staffordshire and, although they were undecorated at first, by 1837 there was a good selection of blue and white ones available. The rate of flow of the milk was controlled by placing a thumb over the hole in the top. Hand-made glass bottles of similar shape were introduced in the first quarter of the century and had the advantage that one could see when they were clean. Later on, moulded bottles, which were much cheaper to make, captured the market. Most had a flattened circular body from which a rubber tube led to the teat. Although long-handled brushes were supplied, the rubber tubes were very difficult to clean — a fact that caused much criticism and gave them the nickname of 'killer bottles'. India rubber teats made their appearance in the 1840s and soon replaced those of cotton or wash-leather and the preserved cows' teats previously used.

Shields were used when the nipple became too sore for a breast-fed infant to be suckled directly. Previously, perforated shields of silver, pewter, ivory and wood had been in use, but most Victorian examples are of hand-made glass. These were fitted with a teat and bone shield or, in the case of those which are curved, with a rubber tube to which the teat and shield were attached. Another method of dealing with the problem was to extract milk from the breast by means of a *breast reliever* or pump and transfer it to a pap boat or feeding bottle. Instead of passing through a teat the milk was drawn into a reservoir by means of a rubber tube with glass mouthpiece, a rubber bulb, or occasionally a piston-operated pump with a valve. They were also used to remove surplus milk, and it was not unknown for a poor mother to feed her own baby on pap so that she could sell her milk to a mother with more money but insufficient milk to feed her child.

Glass *fly traps* were used in the sickroom. They were baited with sugar and water, which was placed in the ring near the base. Flies which entered between the feet of the trap were unable to find their way out again and drowned in the sugar solution. Originally they were fitted with glass peg stoppers, but many of these have been lost and replaced by ill fitting ground glass stoppers or corks.

Breast relievers and nipple shield. (Left to right) Breast reliever (rubber tube and glass mouthpiece missing); cased reliever with piston-operated pump; glass nipple shield.

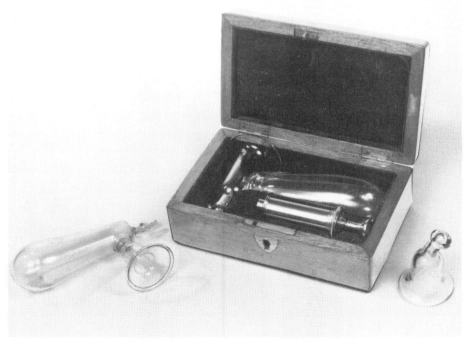

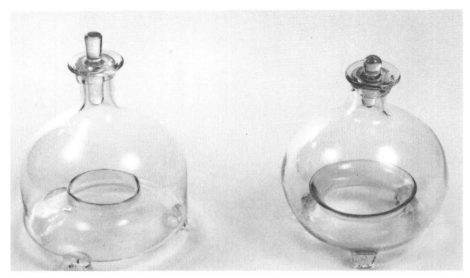

ABOVE: *Glass fly traps.*

BELOW: *Potain's aspirator; wooden monaural stethoscopes; delivery forceps; trephine; case of catheters.*

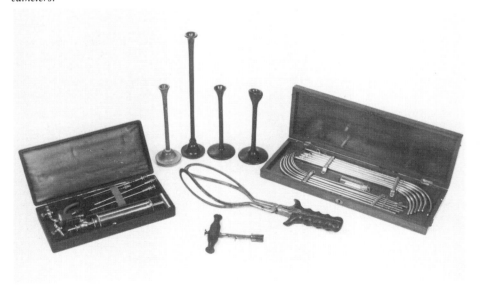

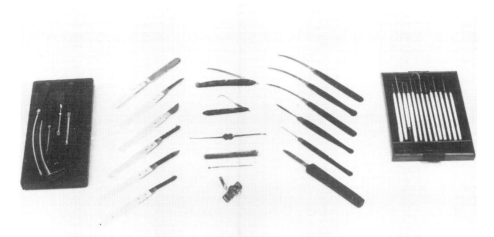

(Left to right) Three straight trochars and one curved one, with chequered ebony grips; curved silver cannula; chiropody instruments with ivory handles; bistoury and tenaculum with tortoiseshell guards; silver lachrymal probe; eye spoon with case and tracheotomy tube; bistouries, tenotomy knives and scalpels with ebony handles; eye instruments with bone handles.

DOCTORS' INSTRUMENTS

The medical and surgical equipment which was supplied to doctors is a very large and specialised field, but some guidelines may prove useful to the would-be collector.

After the introduction of antisepsis by Joseph Lister in 1867, the need to sterilise instruments was slowly acknowledged, and during the next thirty years metal gradually became the accepted material for handles which had traditionally been made from wood, tortoiseshell, ivory or mother-of-pearl. Although most instruments are now made from stainless steel, basic designs have changed little, and nearly all the Victorian specimens to be found can be readily identified from modern instrument catalogues. Many bear the names of well known makers such as Allen and Hanbury, Cox, Evans, Ferris, Maw and Weiss. Silver was sometimes used for items such as probes, catheters, cannulae and tracheotomy tubes, its particular merit being that it would not rust. Many of the smaller objects are not hallmarked. Binaural stethoscopes were patented in 1855, but few examples from the nineteenth century have survived. However, monaural wooden stethoscopes are not uncommon, cedar, boxwood and ebony being the woods usually employed in their manufacture. The long one illustrated was made for a doctor who practised in a poor area of Manchester, its purpose being to keep him as far from his patients' fleas as possible.

Hospitals were smaller and fewer than they are now, and general practitioners frequently performed operations on the kitchen table. Many of the instruments used still lie neglected in doctors' surgeries, and a number of those in my collection have come from this source. I am sure that there are many more still to be found.

FURTHER READING

Bennion, Elisabeth. *Antique Medical Instruments*. Philip Wilson Publishers Limited (for Sotheby Parke Bernet Publications), 1979.

Crellin, J. K. *Medical Ceramics, Volume 1*. The Wellcome Institute of the History of Medicine, 1969.

Matthews, Leslie G. *Antiques of the Pharmacy*. G. Bell and Sons, 1971.

PLACES TO VISIT

Abbey House Museum, Kirkstall, Leeds. Telephone: Leeds (0532) 755821.

Blists Hill Open Air Museum, Coalport Road, Madeley, Telford, Shropshire. Telephone: Telford (0952) 586063/583003.

Brewhouse Yard Museum, Castle Boulevard, Nottingham. Telephone: Nottingham (0602) 411881.

Cambridge and County Folk Museum, 2/3 Castle Street, Cambridge CB3 0AQ. Telephone: Cambridge (0223) 355159.

Castle Museum, York. Telephone: York (0904) 53611.

City Museum, Hatfield Road, St Albans, Hertfordshire AL1 3RR. Telephone: St Albans (0727) 56679.

Flambards Victorian Village at the Aero Park, Helston, Cornwall. Telephone: Helston (0326) 574549/573404.

Jersey Museum, 9 Pier Road, St Helier, Jersey. Telephone: Jersey (0534) 75940.

Museum of Lakeland Life and Industry, Abbott Hall, Kendal, Cumbria LA9 5AL. Telephone: Kendal (0539) 22464.

Museum of Lincolnshire Life, The Old Barracks, Burton Road, Lincoln LN1 3LY. Telephone: Lincoln (0522) 28448.

Museum of North Craven Life, Settle, North Yorkshire. Telephone: Clapham (04685) 414.

Old Kiln Agricultural Museum, Reeds Road, Tilford, Farnham, Surrey GU10 2DL. Telephone: Frensham (025 125) 2300.

Priest's House Museum, Wimborne Minster, Dorset. Telephone: Wimborne (0202) 882533.

Red House Museum, Quay Road, Christchurch, Dorset BH23 1BU. Telephone: Christchurch (0202) 482860.

Ryedale Folk Museum, Hutton le Hole, North Yorkshire YO6 6UA. Telephone: Lastingham (075 15) 367.

Salford Museum and Art Gallery, Peel Park, Salford. Telephone: 061-736 2649.

The Ulster American Folk Park, Mellon Road, Castletown, Omagh, County Tyrone BT78 5QY, Northern Ireland. Telephone: Omagh (0662) 3292.

Warwickshire Museum, Market Place, Warwick. Telephone: Warwick (0926) 43431.

Wigan Pier, Wigan, Lancashire WN3 4EU. Telephone: Wigan (0942) 323666.

Wilberforce House, 25 High Street, Hull. Telephone: Hull (0482) 223111.

Winchester City Museum, The Square, Winchester. Telephone: Winchester (0962) 63064.

Woolstaplers Hall Museum, Chipping Campden, Gloucestershire. Telephone: Evesham (0386) 840289.

Worcester City Museum and Art Gallery, Foregate Street, Worcester. Telephone: Worcester (0905) 25371.

Fort Worth Museum of Science and History, 1501 Montgomery Street, Fort Worth, Texas, 76107, USA.